Superstar of Nicotine Support

Superstar of Nicotine Support

Table Of Contents

Foreword

Among the strongest indicators that nicotine from smoking is addictive is the difference between individuals' desire to quit and stopping success rates. Surveys have demonstrated that the majority of smokers — approximately 70% — wish to quit smoking, yet the successful stop rate stays very low. Get all the info you need here.

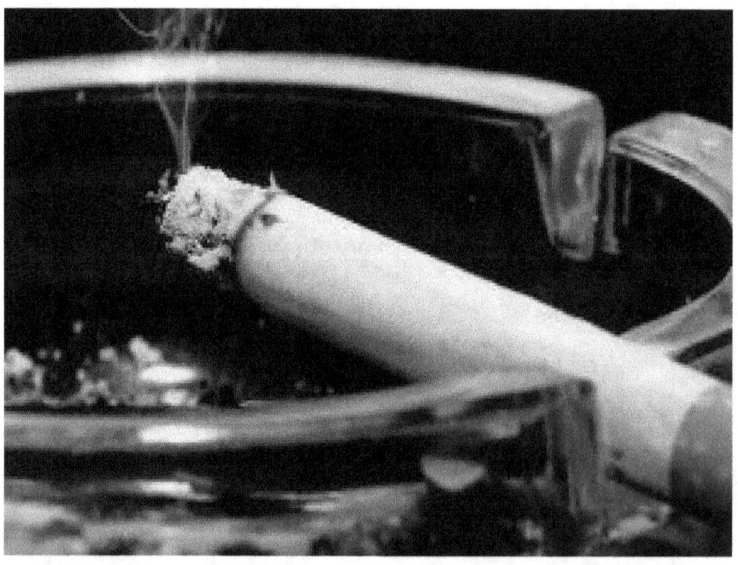

Nicotine Support Superstar

A Look At Counseling And Support Groups For Nicotine Abuse

Chapter 1:

Nicotine Addiction Basics

Synopsis

Read the lists below to acquire a full understanding of smoking and its effects.

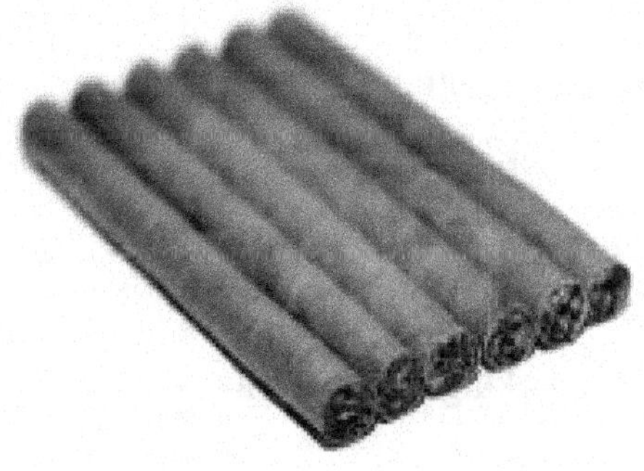

The Basics

All about smoking

Smoking addiction is stronger and lasts longer than most individuals realize as smoking alters the structure and function of your brain.

For some individuals, smoking could be as addictive as cocaine or heroin.

Smoking causes a release of dopamine into the brain, resulting in feelings of joy. Heroin and "crack" have the same forces on the brain.

If a typical pack-a-day smoker takes ten "hits" off each cigarette, that's two hundred "hits" of smoking to the brain every day.

Over time, more smoking is needed to reach the same level of joy. If the brain stops getting the smoking it wants, you'll feel desperate cravings that are hard to overcome with willpower alone.

If a hundred individuals experiment with alcohol or cocaine, about fifteen will become addicted; if a hundred individuals experiment with smoking, about thirty-two will get addicted.

Number of times "addiction" is listed on compulsory cigarette warnings in the U.S.:

Smoking habit

Smoking habits go on the far side of smoking addiction to include individuals, places, and activities, things around us and even moods that are affiliated with tobacco use. These affiliations act together with smoking addiction to reinforce dependence on tobacco.

Smoking withdrawal cravings don't end after you've smoked your last cigarette. They escalate because of your smoking habit addiction.

Once you beat the brain's physical smoking addiction, you've a much better chance of quenching your smoking habit.

Tobacco dependence and its major factor, smoking dependence, are progressive, chronic medical disorders similar to dependence on other addictive substances.

Stopping smoking

A study determined over 90% of those who tried to quit "cold turkey" were smoking again inside six months.

Quitters need to confront both the physical addiction and smoking habit to have the fullest chance of stopping for good.

Smoking Replacement Therapy (NRT) relieves smoking cravings and could double your chances of success.

Americans are four times more likely to try to kick the habit as of the accessibility of smoking patches, gums and inhalers.

The more intensively you center on quitting, the higher your odds of quitting.

 The more techniques you use to quit, the higher your odds of keeping off smokes.

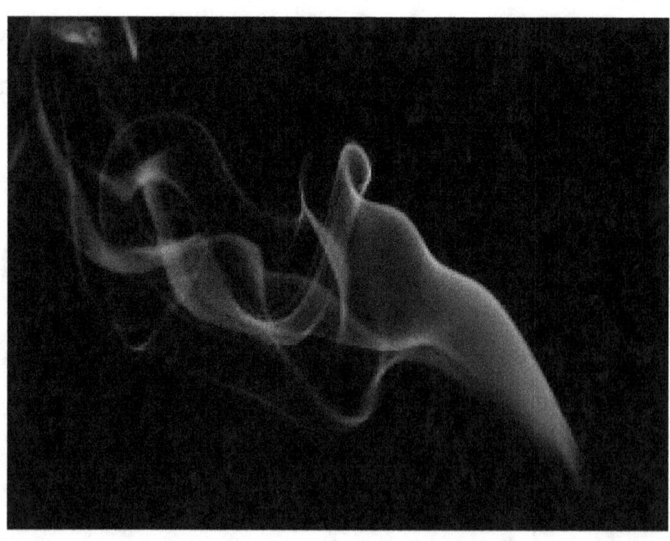

Chapter 2:

Synopsis

We will spare you the lecture. Tobacco use is the head cause of preventable death in the U.S. Left unchecked, smoking might kill more than a billion individuals this century. That equals the number who'd die if a Titanic sank every twenty-four minutes for the following 100 years.

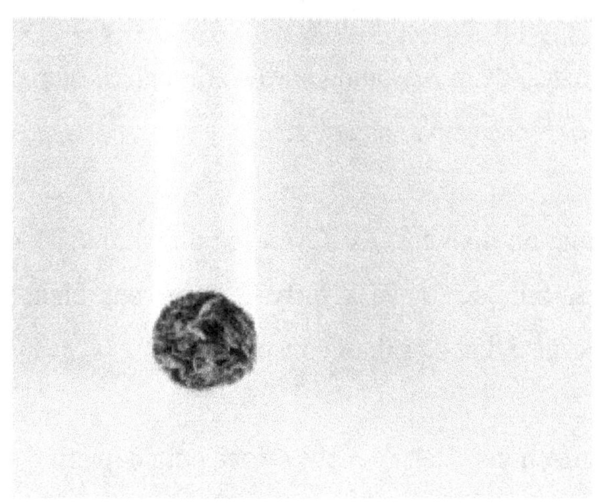

Getting Help

Yet, it might be harder than ever to quit: Three quarters of today's tobacco users attempting to shed the habit are heavily hooked on nicotine, up thirty-two percent from almost 20 years ago.

So quitting, for most, isn't simply a matter of self-control. Even so, the reasons to do so keep accumulating—and they're not all about cardiopathy, lung cancer, or respiratory issues. Here's a few downsides you may not have thought of.

It fogs the brain. Smoking might cloud the brain, according to amassing research. Smoking in middle age is associated to memory issues and to a slide in reasoning powers, though these risks appeared decreased for those who'd long quit.

It might bring on diabetes. As if we need any more risk components for diabetes. Smokers have a forty-four percent higher chance of developing type 2 diabetes than nonsmokers.

It asks in infections. There's really strong data depicting that the risk of infection by pneumonia-causing bacteria is considerably greater for smokers than for nonsmokers.

It may cripple a sex life. A study tracked Chinese men with low risk for arthrosclerosis, and found that smoking might independently hike a man's chance of having a sexual condition.

It might lead to wrinkles...everywhere. Not only does smoking contribute to premature facial wrinkles, but it could also lead to wrinkling of skin that rarely sees the light of day.

It might hurry menopause.

It might dull vision.

It damages bones. Smoking weakens the body's bones and is a serious risk factor for osteoporosis.

Cigarettes can rough up the gastrointestinal system, leading to heartburn, peptic ulcers, and possibly gallstones.

It may stifle sleep. Feeling groggy despite a night's sleep may be an issue for those who light up.

Whether you're ready to quit or just toying with it, call 1-800-QUIT NOW for free support with a trained counselor.

When you call, a friendly staff individual will offer a choice of free of charge services, including mailed self-help literature, a referral list of additional programs in your community, and one-one-counseling over the phone.

A different quit line is the National Cancer Institute's Smoking Quitline, 1-877-44U-Quit, which likewise offers proactive counseling by trained personnel.

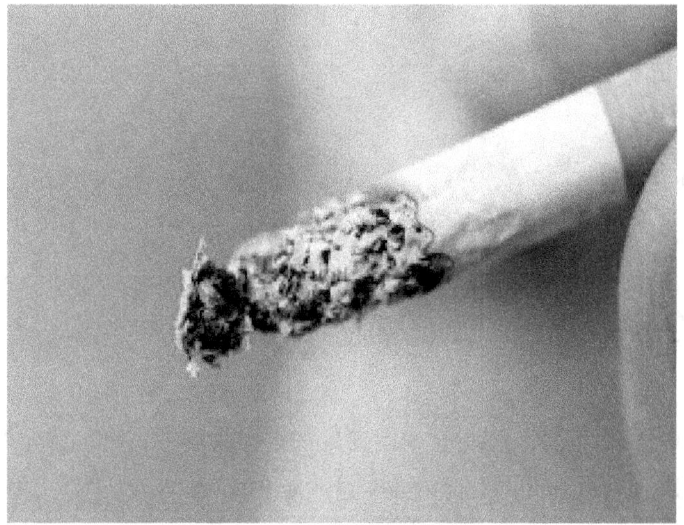

Chapter 3:
Quit Smoking Social Sites

Synopsis

Fresh research has demonstrated that you're more likely to stop smoking if individuals in your social network are likewise attempting to stop the habit at the same time.

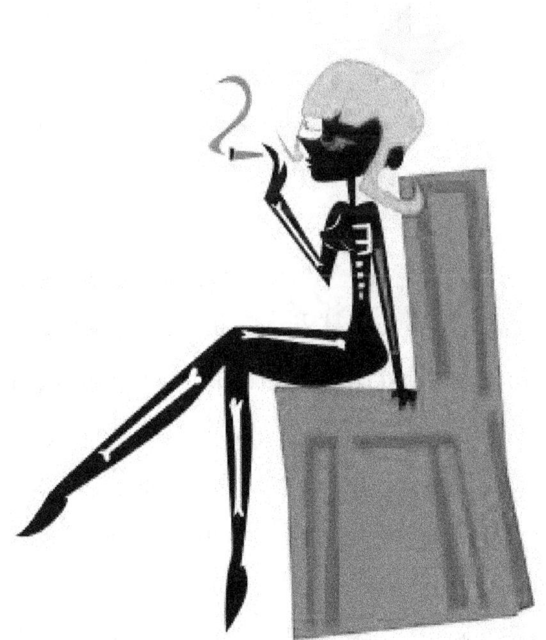

Group Affects

Researchers examined changes in smoking conduct for years in a big social network of 12,067 densely interlinked individuals.

The researchers previously conducted research into how obesity is catching in social networks. Their fresh research determined that the closer relationships are likely to have more influence if one individual is attempting to stop smoking.

Broadly, the researchers ascertained, the closer the relationship between contacts, the bigger the influence if one individual stopped smoking. If one spouse quit, for instance, the other spouse's chances of going on to smoke diminished by 67 %.

Among acquaintances, the effect was 36 %. Among colleagues in small firms, 34 %. Among siblings, the effect was 25 %. Neighbors didn't seem to be molded by one another's smoking habits.

So what might this mean if you run your own social network, discussion board or community blog? If you've a clear aim of something you'd like to achieve, then a combination of shared goals and peer pressure inside closely affiliated groups might help you accomplish your goals.

Amazingly, individuals quit roughly in tandem, with whole groups becoming nonsmokers. Those who went forward to smoke, meanwhile, formed their own "cliques" that, over time, switched from the center of the social network to the outer boundary.

If you have a bigger site, then setting up littler sub groups might help build closer relationships between individuals. For instance, if you run an environmental blog or community web site then you might center your energy on actionable and accomplishable goals, like recycling.

In essence, little closely connected groups will result in behavioral changes. Little groups working together on your site might then shape their own family members and house-mates to alter their own recycling behavior.

Naturally there have been mass anti-smoking campaigns and these might have likewise contributed to the decline in the number of smokers.

The report likewise indicates that education may likewise play a factor in reducing the number of smokers. Centering too much on one certain outcome might likewise alienate individuals and force them to form their own sub-groups.

Those who went forward to smoke, meanwhile, forged their own "cliques" that, over time, switched from the center of the social network to the outer boundary.

Chapter 4:

Face To Face Support Groups

Synopsis

Whether you're an adolescent smoker or a lifetime pack-a-day smoker, stopping might be hard. However with the correct game plan tailored to your needs, you may replace your smoking habits, handle your cravings, and join the 1000000s of individuals who have kicked the habit for good.

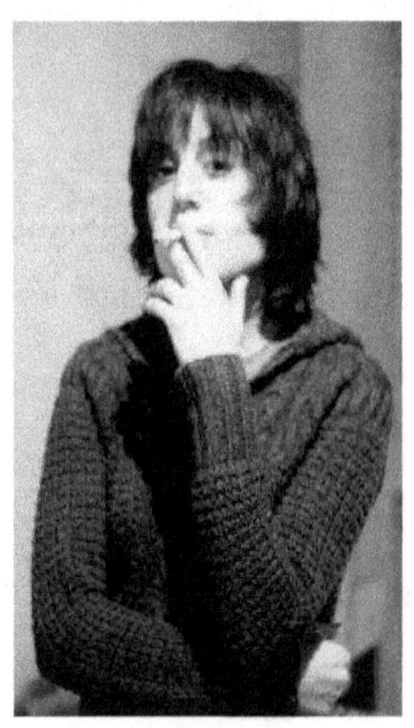

Talking To People

Smoking tobacco is both a psychological habit and a physical dependency. The act of smoking is deep-rooted as a daily ritual and, at the same time, the nicotine from smokes supplies a temporary, and addictive, high.

Doing away with that regular fix of nicotine will cause your body to go through physical withdrawal symptoms and cravings. To successfully stop smoking, you'll have to address both the habit and the addiction by altering your behavior and dealing with nicotine withdrawal symptoms.

Some of the times, it truly helps to talk to soul in person. Giving up smoking isn't simple, and it pays to get good advice to help you as you try to stop.

By discovering the one to suit you, you'll have a greater chance of success.

A supportive group

Support groups are run by experienced consultants, who are trained in assisting smokers to quit. Fixed groups commonly take place over a number of weeks, with a weekly 1 hour sitting. Rolling groups are drop by sessions, with attendees deciding when they show up.

Individual support

One-to-one support is likewise an option. Sessions lasting at the least 20 minutes take place every week over a number of weeks. Remember, you may always discover what's available, and what could suit you best, by calling Smokeline.

It's crucial to remember that you can't make a friend or loved one stop smoking; the decision has to be theirs. However if they do make the decision to quit smoking, you may provide support and encouragement and attempt to ease the tension of quitting.

Look into the different treatment choices available and talk them through with the smoker; simply be heedful never to preach or judge. You may likewise assist a smoker to overcome cravings by engaging in other activities with him or her, and by keeping smoking substitutes, like gum and candy, on hand.

If a loved one slips or lapses, don't make them feel guilty. Compliment them on the time they went without smoking and promote them to try again. Many smokers need several attempts to successfully stop for good.

Many smokers try their first cigarette around the age of 11, and several are addicted by the time they turn 14. This may be worrying parents or guardians, but it's crucial to appreciate the unique challenges and peer pressure teens face when it concerns quitting smoking. While the decision to stop has to come from the teen smoker him- or herself, there are yet plenty of ways for you to assist.

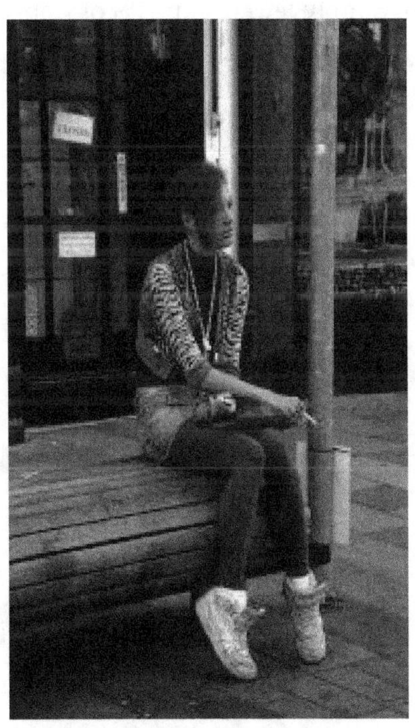

Chapter 5:

Synopsis

In patient treatment may be a big help for smokers who are attempting to quit. Simply fewer than 11% of smokers are able to stop without some type of therapy, according to the latest guideposts.

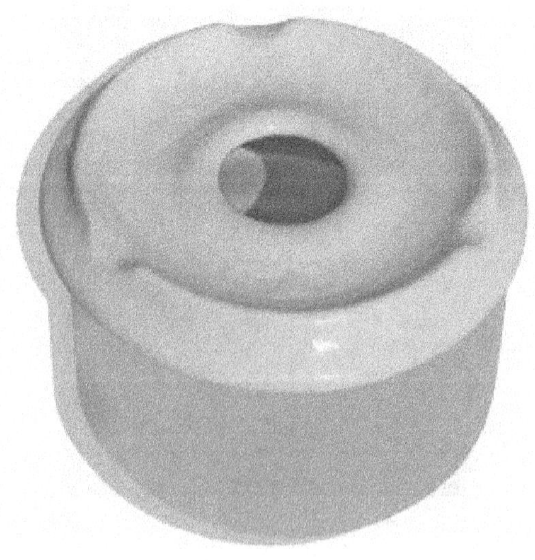

Treatment

However person-to-person treatment (which is found in inpatient care) increases the average success rate to about 17%.

Surely, medication is effective at checking withdrawal symptoms. However it still takes a good deal of effort and behavior therapy to stop smoking.

Though studies found that group psychotherapy and phone treatment step-up success rates, experts state that those methods can't compare to a one-on-one session that's tailored specifically to every patient.

In patient therapy is much more beneficial. Patients need a plan that's customized simply for them. That's something you can't get on the Net or phone.

Person-to-person therapy is helpful for smokers who feel uncomfortable opening up in a group setting. It's simply like a doctor's visit. They don't have to fret about their pride and they may openly vocalize their frustrations.

That was surely the case with one patient. Her in patient therapy session was instrumental in assisting her to quit. "I had too much pride to go to treatment when I had attempted to quit in the past—

I invited to do it on my own," she says. "However treatment was truly what I needed. It helped me recognize what behaviors and patterns were causing me to need cigarettes."

What occurs at an inpatient treatment session?

It's hard to know precisely what to expect in a person-to-person session. There isn't a one-size-fits-all plan.

As a whole, the first order of business is commonly to agree on a stop date and discuss how to brace oneself for it. We discuss how crucial it is to get rid of all cigarette stashes, ashtrays, and matches. A few counselors might also suggest informing your acquaintances and loved ones about your decision and enlisting their support.

When a stop date is set, counselors commonly ask smokers to center on the behaviors and stressors that put them at risk of lighting up. One way to accomplish this is to have smokers visually walk through their day and talk about when and where they acquire the urge to smoke. A few counselors might recommend keeping track of this in a diary.

Smoking is an implanted part of smoker's lives. Treatment may help alter that by centering on the situations or emotions that influence individuals to smoke.

Visually going through their day made them realize what actions, like talking on the phone, triggered them to light up. It helps to open eyes.

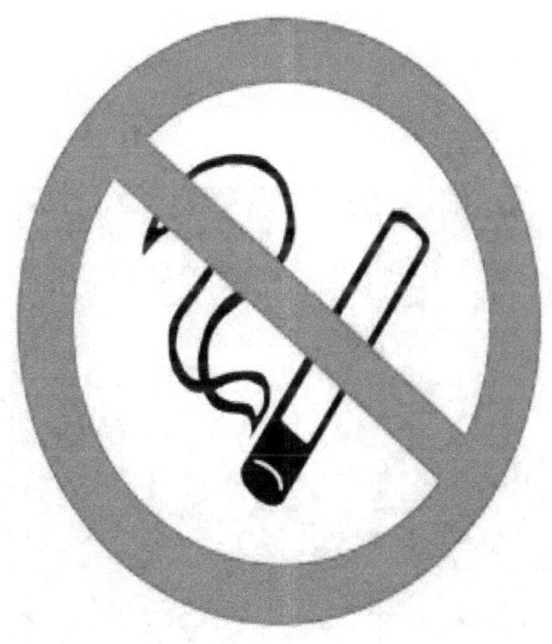

Chapter 6:

The Importance Of Nicotine Education And Prevention

Synopsis

Smoking dependency, like alcohol addiction, is a true mental illness and disease.

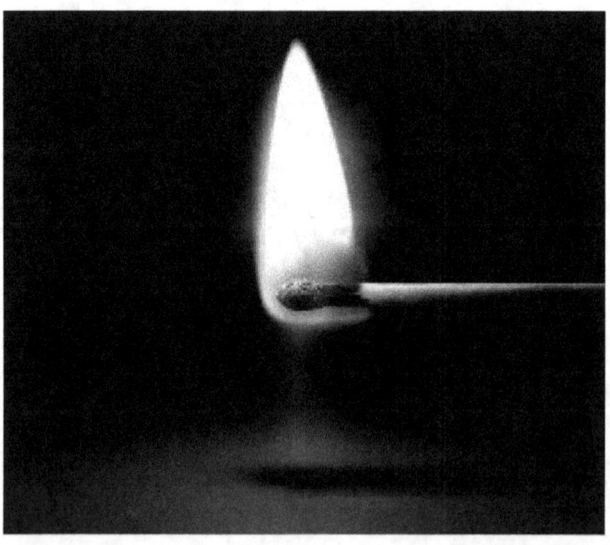

What Is Crucial

While able to totally and comfortably arrest our chemical addiction, there's no cure. It's permanent. Like alcohol addiction there's simply one rule.

Once we are free, just one, using only once and we have to go back. You see, it isn't a matter of how much self-command we have, but how the brain's priorities teacher teaches, how nerve and remembering cell highways that recorded years of smoking have left each of us wired for backsliding.

So why are a few individuals, social smokers, able to take it or leave it, while the rest of us became hooked? Called "chippers," they plausibly account for less than ten percent of all smokers. Envious? If so and still using don't fret, it's normal. That's what enslaved minds tend to dream about, to wish to become like them, to command what for us is unmanageable.

Being immune to addiction is believed to at least in part be related to genetic science. However with up to 90% of daily users hooked solid, spending 1000000s studying smoking dependency genetics is nearly laughable.

Before feeling too sorry for yourself, think what it's like to be an alcohol-dependent and forced to watch roughly ninety percent of drinkers do something that you yourself can't, to turn and walk away. We only have to watch the ten percent who are chippers.

Then again, we were each once chippers also, at least for our first couple of smokes or oral tobacco uses. There was no impulse, desire, crave, hunger or desiring for those first couple of cigarettes. Smoking stimulated our nervous system without our brain soliciting us to come back and do it once again.

 There was no dopamine "aha" relief sensation, as nothing was missing and nothing in need of replenishment. However that was about to change.

Many of us became hooked while youngsters or teens. What none of us knew prior to that first hit of nicotine was how highly addictive smoking it was. Roughly twenty-six percent of us began losing control over continued smoking after just 3 to 4 smokes, rising to 44% after smoking 5 to 9.

What we didn't then know was that inside 10 seconds of that very first puff, that up to fifty percent of our brain's dopamine pathway acetylcholine receptors would get occupied by nicotine, or that before finishing that first butt that nicotine would saturate almost all of them.

Wrapping Up

The great news is that it's all a lie, that drug addiction is about living a lie. Its difficult work being an actively feeding drug addict, and comfortable.

The honorable news is that knowledge is power, that we may each grow smarter than our addiction is strong, that total recovery is altogether do-able for all. In point of fact, today there are more ex-smokers in the U.S. than smokers.

You can do it!

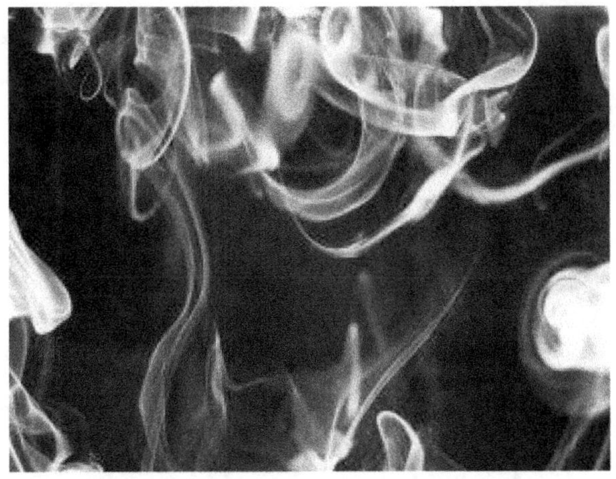